Coronavirus (COVID-19) Variants

What you should know about the variations

Dr. Freeman Morris

Copyright © 2022 by Dr. Freeman Morris

All Rights Reserved.

DISCLAIMER

This book does not offer any medical advice. Should you have any medical issues related to the matter of discussion in this book, kindly/promptly see your doctor. This book is for information purposes only.

TABLE OF CONTENTS

DISCLAIMER 3

INTRODUCTION 6

CHAPTER ONE 8

   What Is a COVID-19 Variant? 8

      What Number of Coronaviruses exist? 9

CHAPTER TWO 12

   What causes new variants? 12

CHAPTER THREE 14

   What Exactly Is the Omicron Variant? 14

CHAPTER FOUR 18

   Other Coronavirus Mutations 18

CHAPTER FIVE 28

   Earlier Coronavirus Variants 28

      What to Expect 29

CHAPTER SIX 32

   Resources to Combat COVID-19 32

Vaccines 32

Masks 33

Testing 34

INTRODUCTION

The virus causing COVID-19 changes continually due to mutation, and new virus variants are anticipated due to these mutations. New variants appear and vanish from time to time. At times, however, new variants linger. New variants will emerge in the future as well. During this pandemic, innumerable variants of the virus causing COVID-19 are being recorded in the United States and around the world.

As a result, the CDC and some other public health agencies are keeping a close eye on all variants of the virus that causes COVID-19 in the United States and around the world.

CHAPTER ONE

What Is a COVID-19 Variant?

Viruses are constantly evolving, which can result in the emergence of a new virus, a new strain, or a variant. In most cases, a variant does not affect how the virus operates. They do, however, occasionally cause it to react in unpredictable ways.

Changes in the virus that causes COVID-19 are being monitored by researchers all over the world. Their findings are assisting experts in determining whether certain COVID-19 variants quickly spread than others, how they may ruin your wellbeing, and how useful various vaccines may be against them.

What Number of Coronaviruses exist?

Coronaviruses did not appear overnight. They are an enormous group of viruses that has existed for a long time. Most of them are capable of causing a wide range of sicknesses, ranging from a minor cough to serious respiratory problems.

COVID-19 is caused by a new (or "novel") coronavirus, one of a few that have been identified as infecting humans. It has most probably existed in animals for a long time. A virus in animals can sometimes infect humans. This is what experts claim occurred here. So, while this virus is not new to the world, it is very new to people. When scientists discovered it was making people sick in 2019, they dubbed it a novel coronavirus. These strains are known as SARS-CoV-2 by experts.

CHAPTER TWO

What causes new variants?

Coronaviruses contain all of their genetic information in form of RNA (ribonucleic acid). Although there are some similarities between RNA and DNA, they are not the same.

When you are infected by viruses, they connect to your cells, enter them, and replicate their RNA, allowing them to spread. The RNA is altered if there is a copying error. Scientists refer to these changes as mutations. These changes occur haphazardly and by chance. It's a natural part of how viruses multiply and spread. Since the changes are sporadic, they may have little to no effect on an individual's health. They can also cause disease at times. For instance, influenza viruses change from year to year, which is why you need a flu shot every year. The flu virus that is circulating this year is not likely to be the same as the one that was prevalent last year.

If a virus undergoes a random mutation that makes it easier to infect humans and spreads, that variant will become more prevalent. In the end, all viruses, which include coronaviruses, can evolve.

CHAPTER THREE

What Exactly Is the Omicron Variant?

The new variant (B.1.1.529) was discovered in Botswana on November 11, 2021, in samples taken. On November 24, 2021, South African experts notified the World Health Organization (WHO) of the Omicron variant for the first time. The variant was unearthed after an upsurge in COVID-19 infections.

Omicron is classified as a "Variant of Concern" by the World Health Organization. This classification indicates that the variant may be more transmissible, cause more severe disease, and be less likely to be receptive to vaccines or treatments. However, more research is necessary to determine these factors. Preliminary evidence suggests that the Omicron variant is associated with a higher risk of reinfection than other variants.

Omicron cases can be detected using current COVID-19 PCR tests. Scientists discovered that one specific PCR test fails to recognize one of the three target genes (dubbed as S gene dropout) in individuals infected with Omicron. As a result, these tests can identify positive Omicron cases and identify this variant more quickly than previous spikes.

Even if you're fully vaccinated, breakthrough infections with the Omicron variant are conceivable, according to studies. COVID-19 vaccines and boosters, on the other hand, remain useful in combating serious illness, hospitalizations, and death. The Omicron variant has surpassed all other strains In the United States. Scientists are closely monitoring how the variant spreads and evolves.

Meanwhile, experts advise getting the vaccine or a booster if you are eligible. Maintain social distance while wearing a mask. If you test positive for COVID or have come into contact with someone who has it, you should isolate yourself for 10 days. If you notice any symptoms, contact your doctor.

CHAPTER FOUR

Other Coronavirus Mutations

❖ **Alpha (B.1.1.7):**

In late 2020, scientists unearthed gene mutations in COVID-19 cases in southeastern England. Other countries, including the United States, have since reported this variant. Scientists estimate that these mutations could increase the virus's transmissibility by up to 70%, allowing it to spread more easily. Some studies have linked this variant to an increased risk of death, but the evidence is weak. The Alpha variant's mutation affects the spike protein, which aids the virus in infecting its host. COVID-19 vaccines are designed to address this issue. Because these vaccines produce antibodies against many different parts of the spike protein, a single new mutation in the

Alpha variant is unlikely to reduce the vaccine's effectiveness.

❖ **Beta (B.1.351):**

Other strains of the virus have been discovered in countries such as South Africa and Nigeria.

The Beta variant seems to spread faster than the original virus and does rarely causes more severe illness.

❖ **Gamma (P.1):**

This COVID-19 variant was discovered in Brazilian travelers to Japan in January 2021, according to scientists and by the end of that month, it had arrived in the United States.

The virus's Gamma variant seems to be more communicable than previous strains. It may also be capable of infecting people who have previously been infected with COVID-19. According to a Brazilian report, a 29-year-old woman contracted this variant following an earlier coronavirus infection a few months prior. Some preliminary research suggests that the variant's changes may help it avoid antibodies that fight the coronavirus (which are produced by your immune system after an infection or vaccination).

According to a laboratory study, the Pfizer-BioNTech vaccine can mitigate against the rapidly spreading Brazil variant. However, additional research is required.

❖ **Delta (B.1.617.2):**

In December 2020, this variant was discovered in India and by mid-April 2021, it has resulted in a massive increase in cases. This extremely infectious variant is now prevalent in 178 countries, such as the United Kingdom,

Australia, the United States, and the entire continent of Europe.

According to a study of the effectiveness COVID-19 vaccine against this variant, it was discovered that:

- After two weeks, two dosages of the Pfizer-BioNTech vaccine were 88 percent effective.
- Two dosages of the AstraZeneca vaccine, which is accessible in the United Kingdom, were found to be 60% effective.
- Three weeks after the initial dose, both vaccines are only 33% effective.

Due to the difference in protection between doses, scientists advise getting the second shot as soon as you are able. According to research, alteration to the spike protein can make the Delta variant up to 50% more communicable than other COVID-19 variants.

The Delta variant of the coronavirus may trigger more serious illness than the previous strain of the virus in individuals who have not received the coronavirus vaccine. People who have been vaccinated may also contract a "breakthrough infection," but they are less likely to become seriously ill or die as a result. The Delta variant has quickly spread and keeps rising given the relatively low vaccination percentage in some parts of the country. The safest way to reduce the spread of the coronavirus and safeguard yourself from severe illness or death is to get the vaccine.

- **Mu (B.1.621):**

This COVID-19 variant (pronounced m'yoo) was first discovered by scientists in Colombia in January 2021. Mu outbreaks have since been reported in countries across South America and Europe.

According to the Centers for Disease Control and Prevention, Mu hit a peak in the United States in June 2021, accounting for less than 5% of variants spreading across the country. It had been steadily declining as of early September. Mu is still being tracked by scientists. According to the World Health Organization (WHO), this variant contains mutations that may make COVID-19 vaccines and our immune systems less effective against it. Preliminary evidence shows it shares some characteristics with the Beta variant, but more research is needed to confirm this.

Mu was identified as a "variant of interest" by the WHO in August 2021. In summary, variants of interest may pose a new risk to global public health, with the ability to spread more quickly, induce more severe disease, or circumvent vaccines or tests. However, they are regarded as less of a risk than "variants of concern," such as Alpha, Beta, Gamma, and Delta. The CDC had not elevated Mu to be a variant of interest in the United States as of September 2021. The agency plan to keep monitoring it alongside the other variants.

❖ **R.1:**

R.1 was discovered for the first time by scientists in some countries, including Japan. In March 2021, an unvaccinated health care worker infected about 45 other employees and residents at a Kentucky nursing home, leading to an outbreak.

In April 2021, the WHO classified it as a "variant under monitoring," implying that some of its character traits may present a risk to humans in the future. The CDC had not classified R.1 as a variant of concern or interest as of October 2021.

Epsilon, Theta, and **Zeta** were once labeled as variants of interest, but the WHO downgraded them. They are still under observation.

CHAPTER FIVE

Earlier Coronavirus Variants

You may have heard that there were multiple strains of the new coronavirus in earlier 2020 when the pandemic was still in its early stages.

A study in China led to the theory about different variants of the novel coronavirus. Researchers were tracking the alteration in coronavirus RNA over time to see how different coronaviruses are related. They examined 103 specimens of the new coronavirus obtained from individuals and also coronaviruses obtained from animals. It was discovered that the coronaviruses discovered in humans were not all the same.

Two types were found, which the researchers referred to as "L" and "S."

They're quite similar, with a few minor differences in each location. The S type appears to have been the first to emerge. However, the researchers claim that the L type was more prevalent early in the outbreak.

What to Expect

- It is plausible that the virus that causes COVID-19 will continue to evolve. New variants may be found by scientists. It's hard to prove how the virus changes will affect what happens. Viruses, on the other hand, are known for their ability to change.
- Reducing the virus's spread by safeguarding yourself and others can help slow the rise of new variants.

- The Omicron variant of the virus that causes COVID-19 infects more individuals and spreads more quickly than the original SARS-CoV-2 strain.
- The Centers for Disease Control and Prevention (CDC) is partnering with state and local public health officials to track the transmission of all variants, which include Omicron.
- Getting vaccinated reduces your chances of becoming seriously ill, being hospitalized, or dying as a result of COVID-19. Keeping your COVID-19 vaccines up to date, including receiving a booster when qualifies, enhances your chances of protection and survival.

CHAPTER SIX

Resources to Combat COVID-19

Vaccines

- COVID-19 vaccination lowers the risk of serious illness, hospitalization, and death.

- People who have received all of their vaccines, which include booster dosage when accessible, are more likely to be protected against COVID-19 variants, such as Omicron. Everyone eligible should get vaccinated and a booster shot, according to the CDC.

Masks

- Put on a mask that fits well, provides adequate protection, and is comfortable for you.

- If you have not received your COVID-19 vaccines and are aged 2 or older, you should wear a mask in public.
- Generally, masks are not required when outdoor. In areas where transmission is massive or high, individuals may decide to wear a mask outside when in close touch with people, especially if
    - ✓ They or somebody they reside with has a compromised immune system or is at higher risk of serious disease.
    - ✓ They have not received COVID-19 vaccines or live with someone who has not received COVID-19 vaccines.

Testing

- COVID-19 tests determine whether or not you are infected at the time of testing. Because it looks for viral infection, this method of testing is called a "viral" test. Examples of the viral test are NAATs (Antigen or Nucleic Acid Amplification Tests).
    - ✓ Additional tests would be required to identify which variant caused your infection, but these are usually not available to the general public.
- As new variants arise, experts will continuously evaluate how well prevailing infections are detected by the test.

- If you have COVID-19 symptoms or have been exposed or may have been exposed to someone who has COVID-19, self-tests may be used.
  - ✓ So when you don't have symptoms and haven't been exposed to someone with COVID-19, using a self-test before assembling indoors with others can provide you with details about the risk of transmitting the COVID-19 virus.

www.ingramcontent.com/pod-product-compliance
Lightning Source LLC
Chambersburg PA
CBHW030045230526
45472CB00005B/1680